ROVING LEADERSHIP
BREAKING THROUGH
THE BOUNDARIES

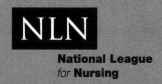

National League
for **Nursing**

ROVING LEADERSHIP
BREAKING THROUGH
THE BOUNDARIES

Salvatore J. Tagliareni, PhD

Janice G. Brewington, PhD, RN, FAAN

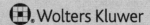 . Wolters Kluwer

Philadelphia · Baltimore · New York · London
Buenos Aires · Hong Kong · Sydney · Tokyo

Executive Editor: Kelley Squazzo
Product Director: Jennifer K. Forestieri
Senior Development Editor: Meredith L. Brittain
Production Project Manager: David Orzechowski
Illustration Coordinator: Jennifer Clements
Manufacturing Coordinator: Karin Duffield
Marketing Manager: Katie Schlesinger
Prepress Vendor: Aptara, Inc.

9 8 7 6 5 4 3 2 1

Printed in The United States of America

Library of Congress Cataloging-in-Publication Data

Names: Brewington, Janice G., author. | Tagliareni, S. J. (Salvatore J.),
  author. | National League for Nursing, issuing body.
Title: Roving leadership : breaking through the boundaries / Salvatore J.
  Tagliareni, Janice G. Brewington.
Description: Philadelphia : Wolters Kluwer ; Washington, DC : National League
  for Nursing, [2018] | Includes bibliographical references.
Identifiers: LCCN 2017030900 | ISBN 9781496396228 (paperback)
Subjects: | MESH: Leadership | Organizational Innovation
Classification: LCC RT89.3 | NLM BF 637.L4 | DDC 362.17/3068—dc23
LC record available at https://lccn.loc.gov/2017030900

DRC0817

*This book is dedicated to my parents, Frances and Sal Tagliareni,
who modeled roving leadership every day of their lives.*
—Salvatore J. Tagliareni

*This book is dedicated in memory of my grandmother, Mrs. Geneva Gilyard.
I give her credit for being my informal mentor, starting when I was around
eight years old. I learned some of my leadership skills from her.*
—Janice G. Brewington

About the Authors

Salvatore J. Tagliareni, PhD is a storyteller, writer, business consultant, art dealer, and former Catholic priest. For over 25 years he has successfully engaged private and public companies in their search for outstanding performance. A gifted speaker, he is blessed with a great sense of humor and can invigorate an audience with insights on life and leadership.

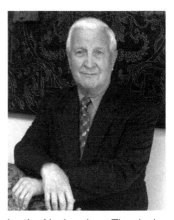

As a young Catholic priest studying theology in Rome, the tragic and unexpected death of his best friend led Salvatore to seek and gain mentorship from Dr. Viktor Frankl, the celebrated psychiatrist and author of *Man's Search for Meaning*. Dr. Frankl and other Holocaust survivors changed the course of Salvatore's life as they shared their personal horrors under the Nazi regime. The desire to humanize the memory of those who perished in the Holocaust was the driving force behind Salvatore's recent novels *Hitler's Priest* and *The Cross or the Swastika.*

After leaving active ministry as an ordained priest in 1973, Salvatore went on to earn a PhD in Leadership and Organizational Behavior and had a successful career as an international business consultant. He is the former president of Next Step Associates, an organizational consulting firm, and for 25 years performed strategic planning and organizational design and implementation for large international companies such as Johnson and Johnson, I.B.M., Hoffman La-Roche, and Boston Financial. He lives in Massachusetts with his wife of 40 years and returns to Europe as often as possible.

Janice G. Brewington, PhD, RN, FAAN is Chief Program Officer and Director for the Center for Transformational Leadership at the National League for Nursing, where she developed and implemented two yearlong leadership programs. She previously served the NLN for three years as chief program officer and senior director for research and professional development. Janice was provost and vice chancellor for academic affairs at North Carolina Agricultural and Technical State University. While at NC A&T State University, she had a unique opportunity to be an "executive on loan" for 18 months with the Gillette Company in Boston, where she was employed as

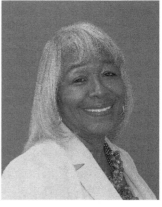

manager for university relations in talent acquisition, human resources, global shared services, North America.

Janice's educational background includes a BSN degree from NC A&T State University, an MSN degree from Emory University, and a PhD degree in Health Policy and Administration from the School of Public Health, with a minor in Organizational Behavior from the School of Business, at the University of North Carolina at Chapel Hill. She also received a certificate from the Management and Leadership Institute at Harvard University.

A fellow in the American Academy of Nursing, Janice has provided organizational development consultation services to nonprofit businesses, city and county agencies, and universities in areas such as organization assessment, strategic planning, team building, effective management, conflict management, coaching, communication systems, leadership, consensus building, and program assessment and evaluation. She also serves as a consultant for numerous group relations conferences in the United States, Europe, and Asia.

Foreword by Former Vice-Chairman of Johnson & Johnson

I first met Sal Tagliareni in the early 1960s. Little did I realize then that this was the beginning of a 50-year friendship and my first exposure to the leadership principles that he lays out so persuasively in this valuable book.

Sal was then a newly ordained Catholic priest and had just been assigned to our parish in New Jersey. He arrived at a time of great change and challenge to the Catholic Church. The Papal council, known as Vatican II, had recently concluded with a virtual tidal wave of changes imposed on the traditional practices, rituals, and organizational principles of the institutional Church. Important among these changes was a redefinition of the roles and responsibilities of the laity, both increasing their influence and imposing new responsibilities. These changes were captured in the phrase "the faithful are the Church."

These changes drew a mixed response from the American Catholic Church and from the members of our parish. In general, the more senior members of the laity and the clergy reacted with questions and concerns. The younger members, both laity and clergy, greeted the changes as an opportunity to refresh and progress the path of the institutional Church. As a result, the burden of teaching and instructing the laity on the content and meaning of the changes, and promoting their acceptance, often fell to the younger priests. Sal was among those who embraced this task eagerly, and he brought me, and many of my like-minded fellow parishioners, to an acceptance of our newly defined responsibilities for the fate of the Church in America. In short, he introduced us to what he has now described as Roving Leadership.

I lost track of Sal soon after, as my family moved out of town and my family responsibilities and my professional career demanded more of my time. Sal, too, experienced change as he traded his clerical robes for academic ones. It was more than 10 years before we made contact again. I had just experienced a radical change in career, leaving my job as general counsel for Johnson & Johnson to become president of one of J&J's pharmaceutical subsidiaries. The path from a staff job to a line job was not one I had prepared for, and I knew I needed help. I needed a coach—someone who understood the importance of building a team, understood what it took to create and lead that team, and, most importantly, someone in whom I had confidence and trust. Fortunately, I thought of Sal.

This arrangement was a success, both from a business and a personal standpoint, and the members of my team later went on to greater career success. As a consequence, I brought Sal in on several further occasions as my career found me in added leadership positions. Each time the results were the same.

So, why, from a practitioner's perspective, is the practice of Roving Leadership a valuable principle to understand and embrace? To understand this, one must first grasp how counterintuitive this idea can seem.

One commonly associates leadership with a hierarchical organization, such as the military or large, multinational corporations. General George Patton and Jack Welch are well-recognized examples of leaders of these types of institutions. The modus operandi of these leaders is based on the command-and-control model, where the determinative directions and decisions are made at the top. Those below the top level serve as advisers and executors. But leadership today is much more complex than this.

The very concept of the all-powerful and knowing leader of the business or nonprofit organization, exercising leadership today through the command-and-control method, fails to square with reality. This is aptly described by Professor James O'Toole in his book *Leading Change*, where he says: "How can a ... CEO of a publicly held corporation overcome resistance to change when the CEO's power is constrained by the diverse and conflicting interests of investors, board members, union chiefs, environmentalists, government regulators, and careerist fellow managers, all intent on marching to the beat of their own drummer?"

An answer to this question, I believe, can be found in the recognition, promulgation, and practice of Roving Leadership. That is why I recommend this insightful and practical book as a valuable addition to the discussion of organizational leadership today.

David E. Collins
Former Vice-Chairman, Johnson & Johnson

Foreword by CEO of the National League for Nursing

This book is the result of an amazing partnership between Janice Brewington and Sal Tagliareni. If Sal is the embodiment of Roving Leadership, Janice is the essence of Breaking Boundaries, and in some profound way they carry both roles together. But who is Janice Brewington?

I read with awe [in the previous foreword] about the growth of the friendship and respect developed over time between David and Sal. So it is with gratitude and pleasure that I have the opportunity to introduce to some, and present to others, Dr. Janice Brewington. I would like to share my perspective of her that shapes and forms this book for leaders who not only break boundaries but can identify their role in managing the boundaries required for transactions within and across complex systems.

Growing up in segregated North Carolina, Janice was influenced strongly by her grandmother, who believed that Janice was destined to make a difference in the world. Janice attended all-black schools for both elementary and high school as well as college. Some might think these circumstances limited her ability to thrive in the bigger, less segregated, but more complicated world. However, at a young age, Janice was identified as an old soul whose wisdom, courage, and authenticity were evident as she coached others to succeed. She dazzled many of all ages, races, and professions with her warmth and her joy in building and sustaining relationships. In other words, Janice broke through the boundaries of segregation to become an example of how a person, community, or institution can refuse to be defined by a system in the minds of other people with stereotypical vision.

Having received her first degree from North Carolina Agricultural and Technical State University (NCATSU) School of Nursing, Janice graduated from Emory University with a master's degree in nursing and later worked as a pediatric nurse practitioner. Later she graduated from the North Carolina flagship institution, the University of North Carolina at Chapel Hill, where she received a doctorate in Health Policy and Administration from the School of Public Health, with a minor in organization behavior from the School of Business. Janice never had encountered a wall that she couldn't find the door to walk through. Boundaries in her mind were meant to be explored, challenged as needed, and used intentionally as markers to enhance the journey.

I met Janice in my role as dean of nursing at NCATSU, and fortunately I hired her as my associate dean. We worked together for more than 10 years rebuilding the School of Nursing where she had begun her professional journey as an academician and clinician. The coaching she started as a child was honed by time, experience, and a brilliant mind, and was used to move faculty from the title of Ms. and Mr. to Dr.

Janice did not limit her coaching to faculty. She co-created leadership programs not only for nursing students but for students throughout the campus. And she pierced the boundary between the academic and corporate worlds as she transitioned, as an executive on loan to Gillette Headquarters in Boston, as their manager for university relations, in the Department of Human Resources, Global Shared Services for North America.

By this time, I was watching my boundary-breaking colleague from afar. We remained friends as she became associate vice chancellor for institutional planning, assessment, and research at NCATSU and moved ultimately to the role of provost and vice chancellor for academic affairs. My goodness, her grandmother's vision was so accurate. Janice was making a difference in the world.

Along the way, perhaps one of the most critical boundaries Janice negotiated was into the world of organizational behavior, working experientially in the Tavistock tradition with small, medium, and large groups. This work centers on boundaries and those who are authorized to use their power to maintain or break the boundary. As one of the few nurses trained, authorized, and treasured as an expert consultant in this work, Janice has crossed international boundaries, working with individuals in Europe and from places as far away as Australia. The lived experience of leading and working with others has strengthened the hurricane force that is Janice.

Now, Janice guides the Center for Transformational Leadership at the National League for Nursing. Dedicated to excellence and co-creating and implementing transformative strategies with daring ingenuity, Janice continues breaking boundaries. This book, co-created with Sal, is a reflection of her courage, leadership, and the role of an authentic truth teller.

Beverly Malone, PhD, RN, FAAN
CEO, National League for Nursing

Preface

What does it take for someone to become a leader? Is it possible for everyone to at times assume the role of leader? What are the beliefs about leadership that stand in the way? What is the path to becoming a leader? What boundaries exist that can impact leadership positively or negatively?

These were some of the questions we asked ourselves when we decided to write this book. As we progressed, we continuously found that more and more questions needed to be answered. Can leadership be taught? Are leaders found only at certain points on the organizational chart? Is diversity an issue in leadership? Are there preferred styles of leadership? Are there specific learning obstacles that, when managed, will promote leadership? Are there learning experiences that can support the ability of everyone to lead?

The result of our questioning is a book that addresses our beliefs about Roving Leadership and the boundaries that must be crossed in order to become a leader. Roving Leadership is based on the empirical evidence that sustained organizational success is not merely the responsibility of one person, or a few persons, at the top. It is not a simple quick fix but a process that utilizes the talents and skills of the entire organization. It helps find the "why" of the organization and provides the energy and skills to positively transform the culture.

This book brings to the reader's attention how leaders collude with organizations to create barriers to taking the authority to lead. Leaders' ability to break through boundaries to lead is also emphasized. It includes amazing stories of individuals who are leaders ... some without a title or position. Through these stories, we dispel the myth that, if you don't have a title or position, you can't be a leader. They demonstrate how the individual becomes self-authorized to lead. Boundaries are presented, and ways to manage boundaries are reflected.

At the end of each chapter of this book is a section titled "Applying Theory to Practice." This section consists of questions or exercises for readers to think about or complete. This book does not offer a "pie in the sky" approach to your becoming a leader; rather, it is based on research and our experiences in literally hundreds of environments. Roving Leadership is a framework for transforming yourself and your organization.

We are aware that on your leadership journey you will face new challenges and that leadership can be messy. We applaud all of you who are willing to push yourselves to a new level of leadership. We hope that in some small way this book will help you fulfill your goals and leadership dreams.

Salvatore J. Tagliareni, PhD
Janice G. Brewington, PhD, RN, FAAN

Acknowledgments

We thank all leaders past and present—those with whom our paths have crossed, those we admire from afar, and those aspiring toward leadership. These individuals provided the impetus for this book.

We would also like to thank Leslie Block for working magic with her excellent editing skills.

Contents

What Is Roving Leadership?

A community is like a ship; everyone ought to be prepared to take the helm.

— Henrik Johan Ibsen

WHY ROVING LEADERSHIP MATTERS

We are proposing a vastly different approach in this book, one that is not based purely on academic literature. Our approach is based on our diverse experiences with corporations, colleges and universities, and the groups for which we had the privilege to serve as consultants. We both have a wealth of experience in academia and with profit and nonprofit organizations.

It has been our conviction, from consistent observation, that many good people are unfulfilled with regard to their careers and work involvement. A great deal of literature indicates that much of this discontent happens because people, by and large, do not feel they are essential and see themselves as part of the maintenance of the organization. We have winners and losers in organizations where the power resides in certain disciplines. There are silos and sandboxes, and it is difficult to grasp that within every organization is the opportunity for everyone to have some sort of leadership position.

If you look at the hierarchy in which many of us were raised with regard to leadership, we tend to think in terms of someone at the top who is all-wise and sees all things clearly. We think of that person as the Wizard of Oz, but as we walk down the yellow brick road of life we realize that no one person has all the skills and knowledge required to be a perfect leader with regard to the hierarchy structure. And a great deal of information is left behind as people do not believe they have been supported with opportunities to become leaders.

There are literally hundreds of definitions of leadership, but we believe that many of them come out of an era that no longer applies in today's complex world. Roving Leadership differs from the traditional view of leadership because it is based on the conviction that sustained personal and organizational success is not really the responsibility of one or a few persons in charge. It is not a quick, simple fix but rather a process that creates positive outcomes by utilizing the skills and talents of the entire organization. The key premise of Roving Leadership is that leadership is not static. It moves depending on the challenges facing the person or the organization. All of the persons and parts of an organization can contribute to this practice.

Roving Leadership positions the organization ahead of the change curve. It allows the organization to find the reason why it exists and provides the energy and inspiration for organizational transformation. Roving Leadership does not depend on the people who have the titles that grant them the "right" to lead. Rather, it is ever-present and takes place spontaneously.

The theory of Roving Leadership is based on the empirical evidence that, with the right circumstances and challenges, everyone can be a leader. Regardless of the environment, there are opportunities for everyone to make a difference. Roving Leadership is a framework for transforming oneself and the organization by widening the concept of leadership and promoting the sharing of power and responsibilities among all those in an organization. Once all members of the organization understand that their contributions are vital, the culture is transformed.

The goal of leadership is not merely to sell ideas, but to enroll others and create value in sharing risks. As leaders we face new ordeals and new challenges, but in this process there will be the development of key strengths and skills. We believe that this will be a change that will benefit the entire organization.

WHAT ARE THE CONDITIONS FOR ROVING LEADERSHIP?

The key premise of Roving Leadership is that leadership is dependent on the challenges the organization faces. All of the members and parts of the organization who contribute to this practice position the organization ahead of the "change" curve.

Roving Leadership exists when the following occurs:

> There is a compelling vision as to why the organization exists.

> Silos are broken down and interdependence is more than rhetoric.

> Strategic direction can come from multiple sources, and not exclusively from within the organization.

> Past success is not taken for granted and does not guarantee future success.

> All persons and units are encouraged to be openly involved in organizational goals and challenges.

> There are no unimportant parts of the organization.

> Belief systems are regularly examined and updated.

> Learning and organizational development are constant.

> Forgiveness is easier to acquire than permission.

> Positive dissatisfaction creates focus for transformational change.

> Failure is a format for learning and adaption, not merely a search for blame.

WHAT ARE THE BENEFITS OF ROVING LEADERSHIP?

In this book we believe that you will discover the following:

> The necessity to authorize yourself as a leader

> The discovery of your individual voice, which will allow you to lead

> That no matter the circumstances, there are always choices

> That speech and beliefs have a great deal of influence over past and current behavior

> That persons and organizations are target oriented and the visuals we create largely determine our behavior
> That habits and comfort zones often prevent growth and change
> That dissatisfaction can be the foundation, both positive and negative, for growth and development
> That leadership does not require a Lone Ranger mentality; there is always a need for mentors and resources
> That measurable goals and plans offer opportunities for exceptional personal and organizational outcomes

ROVING LEADERSHIP CAN BE FOUND IN ALL SORTS OF PLACES AND SETTINGS

There are many myths about leadership that prevent persons and organizations, groups and individuals, from assuming positions of leadership in areas where they have a great deal to contribute. Our observations, in academic circles, corporations, and hospitals, and in the course of our daily lives, indicate to us that leadership is not static; it moves from person to person, dependent on circumstances and challenges. We will address the myths that prevent people from assuming positions of leadership and try to convey the boundaries that stand in the way of assuming positions of leadership.

The stories in this book depict leadership at its best in all types of settings and environments and with myriad individuals. See the following box for examples.

Leadership by an Employee Acting Spontaneously

David was the president of a pharmaceutical company that somewhere along the way acquired a product for coloring eggs for Easter. It was a small product in the portfolio but very profitable. When David was reviewing the mail just before he took a trip to Japan, he found a letter from an angry customer who stated that he and his company had ruined the family's Easter tradition. It seems that the family gathered around to color Easter eggs and the product was defective. In strong language, the writer stated how disappointed she was in the company and the product. David mentioned to his secretary that as soon as he came back from Japan he needed to answer the letter.

When David returned from Japan he was somewhat shocked to find another letter, unbelievably positive, from the same person who had previously criticized the company. His secretary sheepishly told him what had occurred. While David was in Japan, she had gathered every over-the-counter product sold by the company, as well as a dozen roses and a box of candy, and drove a long distance to the home of the woman who had sent the letter. She knocked on the door and profusely apologized for what had happened, hoping that the customer would accept the gifts as a small token of the company's appreciation for her as a customer. The secretary assumed the position of leadership at a moment when it was critical for the company to respond to the legitimate needs of one of its customers.

Leadership by a Faculty Member Who Stimulated Positive Morale

Ethel had become increasingly concerned with the level of negativity of her fellow employees. She decided that she would like to do something to change the avalanche of criticism among her colleagues

---

(*continued*)

and see if there were any positive aspects of working with this faculty. She developed a one-page reflection stating the positive things that she had experienced in her career as a faculty member and posted it on the internal faculty communication board. Initially her comments were ignored, and eventually there were even some very negative comments. However, as time went by, other comments and reflections appeared that indicated there were positive benefits to being part of the faculty. Wisely the dean saw Ethel's reflections and the comments that followed as an opportunity for dialogue among faculty members. The dean's response led to some productive outcomes.

Now, in essence, Ethel had no real understanding of what would transpire, but she had assumed a position of leadership. In doing so she helped create an environment of constructive exchange and mutual understanding of how faculty could work together.

Leadership by an Operator Solving a Complex Manufacturing Challenge

A large company faced a significant operational challenge when it was found that one of its products was decomposing long before the traditional shelf life. It was decided that the company would hire a group of mechanical engineers to study the process. An organizational consultant recommended that the operators of the machines that produced the product be included in the process. The initial reaction from management was, "Why should we include them when it is obviously a mechanical problem that can only be resolved by engineers?" This was a classic example of excluding people based on their position in the organization. It ignored that fact that the experience of the operators could be helpful to the engineers in their search for a solution.

Reluctantly, management agreed to include the operators in the investigative team. Almost immediately one of the operators stated that the machines had been producing a significant amount of condensation, something he had not seen in the past. This seemingly insignificant observation was key to solving what had been a major financial loss for the corporation. The lesson learned is that vital information is not found only at one level of the organization.

Leadership by a Public Servant Preparing for Better Community Relations

Patrolman Joseph never failed to show up early before his shift to cross children through a busy intersection. As the children crossed he would call out their names and playfully model the friendliness and concern of a police officer. When asked by one of the teachers why he was so involved with the children, he responded, "I want those wonderful little children to know from the beginning of their lives that our job is not only to keep them safe but also to let them know that we care about them. If we do our jobs at this level, we are building relationships for the future when they become adolescents and grown-ups."

Leadership by a Promise for Those Who Had Given Up

Sid, a lawyer living in a beautiful community on the Delaware River, was stunned to hear that his community was about to build a sewage disposal plant 600 yards from his lovely neighborhood. There was a great deal of concern and angst on the part of the neighbors, but the overall opinion was, "You can't fight City Hall." Sid stood up at a local meeting of his neighbors and announced, with a great deal of conviction, that the plant would never be built. That bold statement was the foundation for the development of an organization that utilized the many resources in the local community to oppose the proposed plant. It took one year of constant vigilance, but the proposal was defeated. This would never have occurred without the bold leadership that Sid showed at a time when the situation seemed hopeless.

Leadership by a Collective Commitment

Matthew, one of five employees who reported to Edmund, had always been an outstanding performer. But in the last six months his wife had been diagnosed with an inoperable brain cancer, and Matthew was seriously considering taking a leave of absence. Besides the emotional and painful situation of his wife's illness, there was also the consideration that there would be serious financial consequences to taking a leave of absence. Matthew's peers caucused together and proposed a solution that, in many respects, went around the traditional policies of the organization. They asked for a meeting with Edmund and proposed that they could cover all of Matthew's responsibilities when he was unable to fully execute his responsibilities. Matthew's peers realized that this was not traditional policy, but their primary goal was to support Matthew. Edmund wholeheartedly agreed with the strategy. Matthew's wife died while he was on leave, thankful for the remarkable leadership demonstrated by his peers.

Leadership by a Good Samaritan's Witness

One day in the midst of a severe cold spell a man in his thirties sat freezing in a local park. He was wearing only a tee shirt and khakis. Out of nowhere appeared a young woman with a blanket and a cup of Starbucks coffee. She sat down on the bench next to the man and after a few moments draped the blanket over his shoulder and invited him to drink the hot coffee. After a while she picked up his knapsack and invited him to join her in walking across the park to a local church that provided services and hot meals to the homeless. It turned out that the man was a veteran of both Iraq and Afghanistan deployments; he suffered from PTSD. When one of the workers inquired as to why the woman performed so nobly, she replied, "My brother was an Iraq veteran, and after his return he was absent from the family for over two years. He was homeless and we had no idea where he was. One day a Good Samaritan took him to a place where he received services. Fortunately, that was the beginning of his complete rehabilitation. We are once again a whole family thanks to that Good Samaritan, and today was my opportunity to try and help someone else. I had a suspicion that the young man was a veteran and it turned out to be true. Hopefully, today will be the beginning of his being completely restored to his rightful place in society."

Leadership by Living Life Fully Despite Great Tragedy

Jeanne and Chet had five children who all appeared to be healthy, but tragedy struck when their oldest child, at age 8, became blind overnight. This was not the extent of the horror that would invade the life of this beautiful child. For the next 9 years she experienced numerous physical impairments that ended with her premature death. The exact same experience was repeated with two of her brothers. Because of this tragedy, you would imagine that this household would be avoided by most people, but the opposite was true. Jeanne and Chet's household was a magnet, not only for those who desired to help but also for those who considered spending time with them a privilege. There was never a moment when Jeanne and Chet did not understand the pain of the situation, but, somehow, their incredible commitment to life rose above the reality and they chose to make the lives of their children and everyone else around them as fulfilling as possible. Despite their unbelievable situation, they modeled leadership, which enabled everyone in their circle to become better persons.

Leadership by Being a Witness for Social Justice

Mary was a community health faculty member who was involved with a project to offer single-family homes for those living below the poverty line. The location of the project was within the boundaries of a wealthy neighborhood, but one street in particular had been notoriously abused by landlords who provided barely habitable apartments to families without political or social power. The seed money for the homes had been raised by a small group of concerned citizens in a local Catholic church. There was tremendous opposition to the project. Mary attended a key meeting of the town supervisors who would decide if the project should go forward. At one point a citizen stood up and said, "I don't think we should do this because in a short period of time the people in these homes will trash them and they will be eyesores, and I do not think that we should use our taxes in this way." Upon hearing this Mary stood up and said, "As a nurse I have known many clients from this neighborhood who have been keeping

(continued)

your homes clean for decades. I can assure you that they have the capability of caring for their homes in a like manner." Mary's leadership was the turning point and the project was approved.

Leadership by Quiet Compassion

Arlene, age 67, had been diagnosed with breast cancer at age 58 and was being treated with chemotherapy and radiation. She was a spiritual, compassionate person who believed that God was taking her on a journey. She believed that her calling was to minister to others with cancer and shared the small, inspirational books that she enjoyed reading with others. Arlene talked openly with her children, other family members, friends, and even strangers about her cancer. Her friends would often ask her to talk with their friends who were diagnosed with breast cancer, and of course she did.

On days when she took Arlene for chemotherapy treatments at the cancer center, Arlene's niece, Jessica, observed how individuals would gravitate to her aunt and engage in conversations with her about their cancer and how they were doing. It was amazing to Jessica that Arlene could find the strength to minister to others during her own trials and tribulations.

After Arlene completed her therapy, she remained in remission for 8 years. She continued to give others inspirational pamphlets and enjoyed ministering to others in her church and in the community. Arlene and her family participated in activities sponsored by the American Cancer Society, such as the Cancer Walk and Run. She inspired others to explore how they were dealing with their diagnoses and treatment. When her cancer returned, she said that God had prepared her well for the end of life. She had lived her life unselfishly, giving to others.

Leadership by Courageous Intervention

A 25-year-old nurse, Adrian, who worked on the pediatric unit at a major hospital, delivered excellent care to children and their families. Other nurses sought her out to discuss their patients and the patients' family issues. She was innovative in her thinking and ways of delivering care. Assigned to provide care for Natalie, a female infant diagnosed with esophageal fistula, Adrian developed a comprehensive care plan that included the family: a young mother and father, Mr. and Mrs. Mabry, and a 6-year-old brother. Adrian provided education about Natalie's condition and her pending surgery to the parents.

When Natalie had surgery for the esophageal fistula, Adrian was assigned to care for the child. The pediatric surgeon, Dr. Manley, had many conversations with her about Natalie's plan of care while hospitalized and after discharge. Natalie required a gastrostomy tube for feeding, and Adrian demonstrated to Mrs. Mabry how to care for it and how to feed her child. On the day Natalie was discharged, Adrian reviewed the discharge instructions with Mrs. Mabry and told her that she would call the next day to see how she and Natalie were doing. This would also give Mrs. Mabry an opportunity to ask questions.

Over the course of 2 months, Natalie's mother brought her to the emergency room several times because the gastrostomy tube had become dislodged. Several times, Dr. Manley had to enlarge the stricture. As it was noted that the emergency room staff were not sure of the proper protocol for Natalie, Adrian approached the head nurse and offered to write a protocol for ER staff to follow. She also wanted to make home visits to observe how the mother was caring for the gastrostomy and provide more teaching and support. Adrian and the head nurse met with the pediatric surgeon to share these intervention strategies. The surgeon was excited and gave permission for Adrian to proceed with her plan.

With the surgeon's assistance, Adrian wrote a plan for the home visits and an ER protocol that were approved by the pediatric surgeon, head nurse, and the appropriate administrator. As a result of Adrian's interventions, Natalie's trips to the ER decreased, and when she did come to the ER, the staff used the appropriate protocol.

This innovation transpired during a time when hospital nurses did not make home visits after a patient's discharge. During Natalie's teenage years and adulthood, she and her mother would cross paths with Adrian from time to time. Mrs. Mabry expressed how thankful she was for the care Adrian provided for Natalie, especially the home visits.

Leadership by Transforming Leadership

A young administrator at a historically black college and university, Pam continually served as a mentor for nursing students. This seemed to be her calling. Since there were few black students holding office in the National Student Nurses' Association (NSNA) and at state and regional levels, she encouraged her students to run for office. After some coaching, some students wanted to take up the torch, to run for office. Pam provided leadership development sessions during the evening and worked with students in developing and presenting campaign speeches, designing campaigns, and in developing self-confidence. Eventually, four junior and senior nursing students gained the courage and confidence to run for offices.

Pam assisted them to develop winning campaigns. As a result of their leadership preparation, and their ability to become self-authorized to lead, one student was elected president-elect for the NSNA, two became regional coordinators, and one was elected to the NSNA board. One of the inspiring values Pam taught these students was to always reach back and help someone else. As a result, she worked with these leaders to design and conduct leadership development sessions.

The opportunity to lead is all around us. We tend to think of leadership as a series of monumental goals but, in reality, opportunities for leadership exist for all of us in our daily lives. What we do may seem insignificant, but we never know the lasting impact our leadership has on other people.

We are always amazed at the number of people who tell us, years later, that something we said or did had a positive impact on their lives. As you have seen in these examples, Roving Leadership differs from the traditional view of leadership because it is based on the concept that, with the right set of circumstances and the willingness to take a risk, everyone is a leader.

Applying Theory to Practice

- Have you seen examples of Roving Leadership?
- Do you have the desire to become more active as a leader?
- What stands in your way today?
- Why would being a leader have benefit for you?
- Where are the immediate opportunities for you to lead?

2

The Myths of Leadership

The most dangerous leadership myth is that leaders are born—that there is a genetic factor to leadership. This myth asserts that people simply either have certain charismatic qualities or not. That's nonsense; in fact, the opposite is true. Leaders are made rather than born.

—Warren Bennis

WHAT ARE THE MOST COMMON MYTHS ABOUT LEADERSHIP?

One of the key challenges in the search for individual or group leadership is the realization that many of the myths persons and organizations hold about leadership are assumed to be true and are never examined. Some of the most formidable myths that prevent leadership growth and development are as follows:

> *Leadership is innate and cannot be taught.* This is patently false. There are numerous pedagogical and experiential ways to teach leadership successfully. Both the academic literature and the practical experience of organizations indicate that there are evidence-based ways to teach the principles and practices of leadership. We can learn these principles and practices at any age.

> *There are preferred styles that are required for leadership.* There is no single personality style or skillset that is required for leadership. It has been traditionally held that one must be outgoing, verbal, and have exceptional interpersonal skills to be a leader. Yet, shyness does not preclude a person from leading. There are many nonverbal ways to lead.

> *Leadership is dependent on where one finds oneself in the organizational chart.* How often do we hear, "I would love to lead but I am at the bottom of the totem pole in this organization"? Roving Leadership requires action at all levels and does not require a particular title or position on an organizational chart.

> *Leadership precludes women from certain occupations and positions.* Stereotypes continue to exist but they have no foundation in fact. Women are successful in meeting the challenges of leadership.

> *Leadership must always be a top-down reality.* "We must wait until the top of the organization shows us the way" is an old paradigm. Information and opportunity are found at every level of an organization.

> ▸ ***Roving Leadership leads to chaos and confusion.*** "Someone must have absolute authority or it will be chaotic." Clarity of purpose and input from every level do not lead to chaos but, rather, contribute to better outcomes and greater investment in the mission and goals of the organization. This leads to better, more informed decision making and excellent performance.

WHAT ARE THE RISKS OF UNEXAMINED MYTHS?

Many myths are not at the conscious level. However, they influence individuals and the organization as a whole. It has been our experience that myths are held as sacred cows. Although often unspoken, they have behavioral dimensions that indicate to the entire organization that they are true. If it is a hard and fast belief that all significant decisions should be made at the top of the organization, the rest of the organization is, in many respects, immobilized, often waiting for decisions that could have been made at lower levels. If it is a conviction that one must be verbal in order to convey vital information to solve a challenge or problem, then the person who is not verbal but could provide a key element in resolving an issue instinctively takes a backseat.

One of the real dangers in the acceptance of myths is that it implies that there is a preferred, particular style of leadership. This covert message curtails opportunities for those who don't participate in that style of leadership. There is no one style of leadership today that fits everyone. It is imperative to state, over and over again, that leadership is not static and is not found solely within a single style. When the concept of leadership is widened to encompass Roving Leadership, myths weaken, and many people who now are excluded are brought into the process.

The fear that participation at every level will somehow weaken organizational effectiveness by damaging the decision-making process can be readily dismissed. The reality is that no one in any organization has the ability, skills, and charisma to be aware of all of the possibilities that exist before a decision is made. The traditional model of information, which flows from the top down, works to some degree. However, we believe that it curtails the possibility that the organization could function more effectively and have superior outcomes once the flow of information is open to all levels. Roving Leadership does not preclude the reality that, in most cases, there is a group or individual that makes the final decision. Rather, it enhances the probability that the final decision has greater acceptance since those closest to the issue or challenge have significant opportunity to contribute insights and recommendations.

Applying Theory to Practice

- Are you aware of any of these myths in your organization? Do any of these myths affect you in a negative way?
- Are there any additional myths that exist in your organization?
- Is there a preferred style of leadership in your organization? Is that your preferred style of leadership?
- Are any of these myths preventing you from being used effectively as a leader?
- Is your organization open to the concept of Roving Leadership?
- Would Roving Leadership fit with the preferred leadership style in your organization?
- Would rejection of any individual myth be of benefit to your organization?

3

Authentic Leadership: The Real You

When we limit ourselves by being the person we "should" be, we limit our aliveness. We may achieve success but not fulfillment because we are not living out all the important truths about ourselves, truths we need to slow down to excavate.

—Henna Inam

Dr. Jackson demonstrated exemplary leadership as a chancellor. He was an authentic leader and a visionary. He operated on a foundation of core values of integrity, character, and caring. He had the vision for the university to have doctoral programs in engineering and worked across many boundaries to make this a reality. He strategically engaged individuals and groups, such as the governing system of public universities, the vice chancellor for academic affairs, the dean of the college of engineering, faculty, alumni, and the business community in planning for this innovative plan. He created organizational leverage based on the institution's history and track record as an excellent, well-respected university. As a result of his leadership and his ability to recognize the roving leaders within the university, the PhD programs in engineering were approved by the systemwide governing body. Thus, the institution became a doctoral/research intensive university.

Dr. Jackson was passionate about his work at the university and was a strong advocate for ensuring the survival of all academic programs, especially nursing. Just as with engineering, he had a tremendous impact and influence on the success of the school of nursing. He became knowledgeable about all aspects of the school of nursing and familiarized himself with statistical data amassed by the state board of nursing.

Perhaps his greatest legacy as an authentic leader was the special relationship he developed with students and student organizations and the successful leadership forum he created for student leaders. Inspiring students to become leaders was his calling. Because of Dr. Jackson, the university continues to flourish and excel, establishing innovative programs, developing partnerships, and engaging in cutting-edge research.

Authentic leadership has been defined as "a pattern that draws upon and promotes both positive psychological capacities and a positive ethical climate, to foster greater self-awareness, an internalized moral perspective, balanced processing of information, and relational transparency on the part of leaders working with followers, fostering positive self-development" (Walumbwa, Avolio, Gardner, Wernsing, & Peterson, 2008, 94). In life and leadership, we are taken on a journey that stops off on different paths along the way. Some of us believe that God has a plan for us and brings us on this journey, while others have a different vision for life's vicissitudes. Whatever we believe, it is safe to say that there are lessons to be learned as doors open and close. We need a safety net to hold us until it's safe for us to soar. Think of the airplane on the runway. The pilot is in a "holding pattern" until the storm clears and the air traffic controller states that it is once again safe to fly. While on the journey to leadership, we may feel like Alice in Wonderland who says, "I know who I was this morning, but I think I must have changed several times since then" (Carroll, 1865, 2).

How we embrace our authentic leadership makes the difference. As leaders, if you have a foundation of core values that guides who you are as an individual, as a leader, as an authentic leader, you don't have to worry about changing and not knowing who you are. Some aspects about you may change, but your core values should remain the same. As leaders we have to know our North Star, our guiding star—our navigation system.

Your North Star is a compilation of your core values that will help you navigate in systems that may be treacherous or confront those who lack moral fiber. When you're clear about your core values, you can lead with moral courage and integrity and not fall prey to those who do not possess such values.

Sometimes we—especially women—may be asleep within the recesses of our own minds. There is perhaps a fear that when we awaken, there will be a need to harness the boundaries invading our minds and unleash the power and courage that have been dormant. Then the question becomes, Do we have the courage and want to take the risk to embrace this new phenomenon?

The conscious mind says, "Wake up," while the unconscious whispers, "Sleep." To which voice do you listen? Do you listen to the voice that is trying to free you to become your authentic self, or do you listen to the voice of fear that is trying to suppress your authenticity? How can you remove the mask to be the authentic leader you're called to be? The choice is yours.

As leaders, when we are clear about our authentic selves, we can embrace the leadership of others. We engage in collaboration while some may engage in unhealthy competition, failing to value the assets that others bring to the table. For example, just as schools of nursing are integrating interprofessional education into the curricula, health systems are working toward interprofessional practice, to provide quality and safe, coordinated care to patients/clients, families, communities, and populations. When we are clear about who we are as leaders, we can engage in co-creating planning and the coordination of quality and safe care that are key to helping heal the people we serve.

Authentic leaders understand that all members of the team need to be authorized to take up the mantle of leadership in the best interest of the patient/client. When this happens, the power of a team engaged in collective healing is most effective. This is powerful because Roving Leadership is integrated in the system and the team begins to co-create action plans for care coordination. This is truly authentic leadership at its best.

Applying Theory to Practice

- Define your core values.
- Identify ways you integrate your core values in everyday life and in your work.
- Identify three leaders you admire as authentic leaders. What authentic leadership traits do they possess?
- Identify ways you integrate your core values into your leadership.
- What authentic leadership qualities do you have?
- What do you need to change about how you lead?
- What boundaries do you need to overcome?
- What boundaries do you need to maintain?
- Why is it important for you to have permeable boundaries?
- What is your action plan to become the authentic leader you are destined to be?

4

Personal Authorization to Lead:
Why Is Authorization Important?

Too many of us are not living our dreams because we are living our fears.

—Les Brown

Before one can assume the responsibilities of Roving Leadership, it is vital to recognize that there are often boundaries that must be crossed in order to achieve the desired results. It has been our experience that Roving Leadership is not possible until we authorize ourselves with the belief that we are leaders.

In a very real sense, the first decisions we make about ourselves are the result of influences and inputs from others. In childhood many messages are accepted literally, without reflection or understanding, and these have implications for our future behavior. Without attempting to seek out villains in this process, it is important to underline the reality that the first decisions we make about ourselves are, to some degree, flawed. To assume our rightful position as leaders under the proper set of circumstances, it is vital that we consciously make the decision that we are leaders, that we deserve to be respected as leaders, and we have a great deal to offer. We refer to this process as authorizing yourself.

The past is not necessarily a prologue to the future. Certainly we can learn from the past, but to believe that there are no alternatives because of past circumstances and behavior is to freeze options with regard to the present. There are times when we think of ourselves as persons who have difficulty changing when, in fact, the amount of change that happens in all of our lifetimes is mammoth. We make changes every day, based on, for example, new relationships and new career opportunities. We change when it makes sense to change. Without self-authorization, and without the conviction that it is possible to influence outcomes, people resist the change process and fail to see the level of control that exists within it. In that way we become resistant when the change, whatever it is, does not seem to make sense, has too big a price, and has questionable rewards. As leaders, we begin to examine our resistance and what is operating in our "system in the mind" about the fear of changing. Only then can we process and identify the real value in how we want to change and how to assume our authority to be a leader. Those who learn to see that leadership is not foreign to them and beyond the realm of what they consider to be ordinary circumstances will begin consciously to seek out opportunities in which they—and possibly only they—can meet that particular challenge.

It has been our experience that if we do not consciously accept the fact that we are leaders and position ourselves for that important role, we will be largely ignored. The opportunities to contribute in our personal lives, as well as in our careers, will be limited. It is vital to believe that our inner voice is critical and needs to be shared. The concept of self-authorization is not in any way an indication of arrogance, of placing ourselves above others. It is rather a definition of the individual value that each of us brings to a particular set of circumstances.

Authorization of oneself as a leader does not depend on an organizational chart or where we went to school, our age, or other accidental properties. It is based on the conviction that under the proper set of circumstances, anyone can be a leader. We must authorize ourselves as a vital foundation to becoming leaders. There is no need to wait for permission. And previous leadership success is not a prerequisite for current and future success.

Being self-authorized means that you can discover your own personal power to lead and also to help others become self-authorized, to take up their leadership. Sometimes individuals have selective amnesia and forget about their personal power and how they can use it to influence change and transformation.

Applying Theory to Practice

- Can you say the following aloud: "I am a leader and I deserve the opportunity to lead"?
- What does it mean to have your own voice?
- If you had your own voice, what leadership opportunities would you tackle?
- Are there any immediate opportunities for leadership in your personal or professional life?
- What stands in the way?
- What are some of the positive affirmations you would make that would indicate to your brain that you are very serious about taking on the challenge of leadership?
- Are there new beliefs that you would like to substitute for your old limiting beliefs?
- If you were to establish a visual about what you would like to achieve with regard to leadership, what would it look like?
- Give some examples of Roving Leadership that you have experienced in your family, your home, or your organization.
- If you had to select one area in which you could immediately begin to shape or resolve an issue with regard to leadership, what would it be?

5

Understanding the Politics of Organizations

If you're going to kick authority in the teeth, you might as well use two feet.

—Keith Richards

When Dr. Andrews was appointed associate vice chancellor for institutional, planning, assessment, and research, she had to implement a redesign of the unit. As she engaged staff in this process, the issue of the Human Resources System (HRS) kept rising to the top. After engaging in an organizational assessment, she identified the role that two of her divisions had in this process. Then, after compiling more information, she determined that the HRS was not an issue for her area alone but was a systems issue.

The HRS was complex and involved other departments within the university. Dr. Andrews learned that a team had been working on plans for integration of a fully operating HRS for the past two years, but the plan was on hold because no one was leading the process. She identified the individuals and teams from departments that had previously worked on the system (business and finance, information technology, and human resources), and based on her assessment, realized that issues of leadership, authority, power, and competition were operating among the units.

Because of her experience with organizational systems and behavior, Dr. Andrews initiated the following process, which the provost supported. First she scheduled individual meetings with the vice chancellors and directors who supervised team members to inform them of her finding and work with them to co-create a new plan. Having obtained buy-in to lead this initiative, she scheduled a joint meeting with all individuals involved including the project manager and the team leaders from participating departments. The discussion focused on issues, challenges, and reasons why the initiative had stalled with further discussion of roles, boundaries, leadership, authority, power, and competition. Plans for subsequent team meetings ensured that the project manager and team leaders would have leadership roles during the meetings. In the meantime, she conducted individual and group assessments (using valid and reliable instruments) on team functioning, communication, and conflict management. The data were presented to the project manager, team leaders, and team members.

This aspect of the project involved workshops and team building exercises. The project manager and team leaders were assigned the task of developing roles and responsibilities for each team and obtaining input in order to establish reporting responsibilities and accountability. After the HRS system was fully operational and functioning for one year, a celebration was held and the teams were presented with certificates of recognition. This innovation would not have happened without the integration of the concept of Roving Leadership.

Bolman and Deal (2013, 181) define politics as "simply the realistic process of making decisions and allocating resources in a context of scarcity and divergent interests." Politics in organizations is an interesting phenomenon, with many individuals believing that politics do not exist. Such individuals have the illusion that if they just move to another organization, they will leave the "stuff" behind. They do not understand that politics are always alive and well in organizations, and that while names and faces change, the "stuff" remains the same.

The solution for these individuals may not be to leave the organization (unless the environment is toxic), but rather, to learn how to manage the politics of organizational systems. If you understand the dynamics of what's happening in the system—if you can name it and put a label on it—then you can begin to become intentional about developing strategies to address and manage the politics of organizations.

Many have a negative view about politics, especially when an individual takes action to gain power and use it for personal benefit, which is not in the best interest of the organization. However, politics does not have to be negative. How leaders and stakeholders manage the issues of scarce resources and issues related to organizational processes, that is, leadership, authority, power, and competition, can be both positive and negative.

The important phenomenon is how these organizational processes are enacted in the organization. It is important to understand the following key terms:

▸ **Leadership:** Bennis (2009) states that leadership is elusive. He further indicates that leadership is the ability of capturing the vision. Leadership is also about influencing others to buy into a vision for the organization's success. In *Leading Change*, Kotter (2012) indicates that sometimes leadership is thought to be hierarchical with the leaders at the top and others at the bottom level. This isn't true because there is always room for others to lead. This is where Roving Leadership can occur and leadership can be dispersed in the organization.

▸ **Authority:** Authority is the ability to have influence or power over others, especially subordinates in organizations, engaging in decision making and giving direction to subordinates for the purpose of achieving the organization's goals.

▸ **Power:** Power is the ability to have influence over others, for the good of the organization or for personal gain and the detriment of the organization.

▸ **Competition:** Competition is rivalry. In organizations, one may compete for clients, products, market share, or for a position within the organization.

Issues in all these areas happen among individuals and within and across groups in organizations. Any of these issues can become negative. For example, a program coordinator who reports to the newly hired associate dean in a school of nursing has difficulty with authority and leadership and exhibits resistant behavior. He does not complete assignments and is often absent from meetings. When he attends meetings, he fails to support the associate dean's recommendations or ideas. The program coordinator, it seems, had also applied for the associate dean position and is upset because he was not selected. The source of his issues with the associate dean's leadership and authority is competition. He believes he should have been selected for the position and could do a better job.

It is important for leaders to be cognizant of issues of this type and be able to name them and claim them before attempting to intervene. It is essential to address the issue rather than ignore it. In a situation such as this, the associate dean should engage in coaching, giving, and using crucial conversations to address all issues and not pretend they do not exist.

Applying Theory to Practice

- Identify a time within the last month when you experienced an issue with an organizational process (e.g., leadership, authority, power, competition) in your current position.
- Describe the situation/issue.
- Describe what you did about the issue.
- What was the outcome of your action?
- How would you evaluate your results? Was your action(s) successful? Why were your actions successful? If your actions were not successful, what could you have done differently?

6

There Are Always Choices

Don't live life in the past lane.

—Samantha Ettus

IS IT TRUE THAT AT TIMES THERE ARE NO CHOICES?

Jane, age 36, has been with an organization for seven years. An outstanding worker who responds immediately to every task or assignment she is given, Jane has the feeling that she is stuck. She has, in fact, been labeled as one who always comes through but is not promotable. Lately Jane has started to experience a high level of frustration because she feels that she is taken for granted. More and more she gets the feeling that people have been promoted who contribute far less than she does. She is aware that her energy level, which has always been exceptionally high, has been diminished by her belief that there's very little in the future that she can look forward to and that this position offers no option for growth. She is also aware that for at least the last six months, she is taking this level of frustration home and has more and more difficulty separating her personal life from her career. In essence Jane is feeling that there are no viable options for her within the organization.

There are many times in life when we feel we are stuck in a rut and don't have choices. Often we refer to the current situation by saying, "I wish I had some other choices but for a lot of reasons I have to play the hand I was dealt."

We are not going to dismiss this feeling out of hand because it is a genuine feeling. It is so strong and so pervasive that it makes it almost impossible for us to see that there are always alternatives. No one has total control over the circumstances and happenings around them, but it is worthwhile to establish the possibility that no matter the circumstances, there are always alternatives.

This conclusion comes to us through the eyes of Dr. Victor E. Frankl, author of *Man's Search for Meaning* (Frankl, 1959). In the early 1930s, Victor was a successful surgeon and psychiatrist living in Vienna, on the way to becoming one of the foremost psychiatrists in Europe. Trained with the traditional belief that the past primarily determines current and future behavior, Victor established a whole new therapeutic approach that would eventually become a major force in the field of psychiatry. However, just as he was becoming more and more influential, the Nazi party incorporated his beloved Austria into Germany.

21

As a Jew, Victor soon began to suffer the consequences of Hitler's persecution of Jews. In the beginning the restrictions were slight and seemed insignificant, and, like many Jews, he believed that Hitler's form of inhumanity would never take root in his homeland. However, what was perceived to be insignificant became more and more horrific as Victor was stripped of his citizenship and his medical practice was restricted. Eventually he was incarcerated in four successive concentration camps where he suffered every form of human degradation and was, at times, close to death. His father had died in a concentration camp and his mother and his wife Tillie were sent to Auschwitz.

Victor suffered from typhus and malnutrition, with freezing conditions in the winter and appalling heat in the summer and absolutely no control over the circumstances of his life. More than being in a rut, he was in a truly hopeless situation. It is hard to imagine how all the losses he experienced did not completely pulverize his spirit. We can easily understand how he might have given up and allowed himself to wither away.

At one point in his incarceration, however, Victor realized that if he were to concentrate on all that he had lost he would probably have little chance to survive. He realized that there were certain circumstances over which he had absolutely no control—without warning or reason, guards could simply decide to shoot someone. However, he arrived at a point where he realized that he needed to have some way to respond to the fact that while he could not control circumstances, he could control how he responded to them. Tillie, who was to his knowledge still alive, became a driving force in the choices he made. Instead of being immersed in overwhelming feelings of loss, he made the conscious decision that because he believed Tillie was alive, there would come a time when they would be reunited in Vienna. He began to speak to Tillie every day and imagine all of the things that are normal in the course of life, like having a picnic or dancing in Mozart Park. This choice, he maintained, was the reason that he continued to live despite the circumstances.

IS LEADERSHIP POSSIBLE WITHOUT THE BELIEF THAT THERE ARE ALWAYS CHOICES?

In order for leadership to exist, one must believe that there are choices. In fact, denying the possibility of choice is a choice in itself. Leadership can be draining and messy and at times one of the alternatives is to believe that there are no choices. However, it is imperative that despite the circumstances, leaders realize that choices exist. Initially, looking at a situation at the feeling level, it is normal to believe that there is nothing one can do. We might say to ourselves, "I have no choices. I don't have any power to change the situation."

It is common to make the situation even worse by bringing new information to the problem of why we are stuck. The tendency is to invest 90 percent of our energy in making the problem worse than it is. The circumstances become so overwhelming that all we really see is the problem.

The more positive alternative is to recognize that, no matter how dire the circumstances are, there are always choices. It is not initially imperative that we have solutions, but it is important to look at the problem from a different framework. We might ask what it would be like if we didn't have this problem. Leadership requires more than problem definition. When leaders establish what it would be like if they did not have the problem, choices emerge.

Applying Theory to Practice

- Have you ever experienced being in a rut?
- If so, what did it feel like?
- What were the effects of being in this rut?
- Did you believe at the time that there were no alternatives?
- Did you share this situation with anyone?
- What were the most difficult parts of this?
- What steps did you take to get out of the rut?
- If this were to occur today, would you handle it differently?
- Do you believe you have choices regarding opportunities to lead?
- If so, what are some of those choices?

7

Limiting Beliefs and Negative Self-Talk

Whether you believe you can or you can't you are right.

—Henry Ford

HOW DO BELIEFS AT THE CONSCIOUS AND UNCONSCIOUS LEVELS LIMIT LEADERSHIP OPTIONS?

Two boundaries that limit opportunities for leadership are limiting beliefs and negative self-talk; they are interconnected. Limiting beliefs are a reservoir for those negative self-messages that bombard us in our daily lives.

> Muriel, age 42, was raised in a culture where one limiting belief was that it is not ladylike to appear too intelligent in public. Her culture consistently reinforced the notion that if she wished to marry and find happiness, she should present an image of one who is caring but not opinionated. Muriel believes that this foundational belief influences every aspect of her life, especially her career.

Throughout our lives, beliefs influence our behavior, and often we are not conscious of these beliefs. Some are cultural and are assumed early in life, when there is little reflection or understanding of their implications, and they make sense, especially for those who are in the process of modeling a way of life. But the reality is that when we are adults, striving to make significant contributions, both personally and professionally, many truisms become limitations. Although seemingly trite, these beliefs do influence our behavior. For example:

➤ Children should be seen and not heard.

➤ Don't ever blow your own horn; it is not nice and people will not respect you.

➤ It's better to be shy and retiring than to be out in front.

➤ If you present yourself as overly intelligent, people may think that you are arrogant.

➤ If you don't go to certain schools and have certain degrees, then by and large you won't be taken seriously.

➤ Be slow to speak because opinions, once verbalized, can have negative consequences.

➤ There are few people in this world who can become leaders, so be careful about the risks you take.

HOW DOES NEGATIVE SPEECH LIMIT THE OPPORTUNITIES TO LEAD?

Your self-talk is the channel of behavior change.

—Gino Norris

> Frank, age 43, has a consistent habit of speaking negatively to himself. When something happens, instead of saying, "That was difficult. How am I going to deal with it?" he immediately refers to the situation by saying to himself, "This always seems to happen to me. I cannot believe how stupid I was to try this and not look at the consequences. I could kick myself for believing that something was going to be different this time; no matter what I do it always seems to go south."

As in the case of limiting beliefs, negative self-talk can be a serious obstacle that must be challenged. Speech and beliefs often create limitations for leadership, and Frank's behavior, to a large degree, stands in the way of any positive experiences.

It is well known that we speak to ourselves, literally, thousands of times during the day. For some people, a great deal of that speech can be negative, and we know through observation and research that the messages we send ourselves influence our choices, behaviors, attitudes, and outcomes. These messages carry a great deal of weight in the choices that we make: for example, the person who consistently says, "Things never work out for me" will overlook many opportunities to lead. Statements such as the following can be damaging to personal growth as well as to career opportunities:

▶ "I missed my opportunity, and it's too late for me to be a leader in this organization."

▶ "I wish I had a doctorate; I feel that I have the skills, but I'm overlooked."

▶ "I wish I weren't such an introvert. I'd like to take the opportunity to lead, but I'm basically shy."

▶ "If I hadn't made so many mistakes in the past, maybe I would be better positioned to lead."

▶ "Where I am in this organization makes it impossible to be noticed, and so the opportunities to lead are nonexistent."

▶ "I don't think anybody values me enough to see me as a leader."

Because self-talk statements influence the choices we make, it is critical to monitor them. Positive self-talk is not just a bromide—it is a critical requirement of Roving Leadership. Positive statements send signals to the brain, which reinforce the desires and outcomes that lead to the acceptance of leadership opportunities, wherever they emerge within the organization. Positive self-talk assists the ability to reframe negative messages so the messages received by the brain will be more constructive. Reframing (Table 7.1) is a powerful tool for diminishing and altering the effects of negative messaging.

The following are examples of positive self-talk:

▶ "Despite the fact that I'm not perfect, I'm a valuable, skilled human being who deserves to be respected and needed."

▶ "There have already been circumstances in my life where I have been a leader and have done well."

TABLE 7.1

Reframing Negative Self-Talk

Negative Self-Talk	Reframed Self-Talk
"This is too hard, and I'm afraid to try it."	"This is a chance to learn something new."
"The leadership challenge is too complicated."	"I'll break it into manageable pieces."
"I don't have the skills or the resources."	"I'll find a mentor and some allies to assist me."
"I'm overwhelmed, and there is no way I can get this done."	"I couldn't fit it into my schedule, but I can reexamine some priorities."
"I may fail, and I fear that."	"Trying will grow my skills and provide opportunity for growth."
"Now is not the perfect time."	"There is never a perfect time."

➤ "I believe that there are opportunities for me to make significant contributions as a leader."

➤ "Each day I'm becoming more aware of my individual voice and the contributions that I'm making."

➤ "My style of being a leader can be as valuable as any other style."

➤ "I'm not going to be stuck by anything that happened in my past because I believe that now I'm ready, willing, and able to lead."

Applying Theory to Practice

Limiting Beliefs
- Are there any beliefs that negatively influence your ability to lead?
- What feelings accompany these beliefs?
- Do you consciously accept these beliefs?
- Do the beliefs lead to limitations in your life?
- Do you accept these limitations as unchangeable?
- What new beliefs would you like to add?
- What would be their value?
- What would it feel like if you followed the new beliefs?

Negative Self-Talk
- Is negative self-talk part of your daily speech? (Carry a small notepad and periodically list your patterns of self-talk.)
- Are you aware of the negative voice in your head that consistently sends negative messages? (Give that negative voice in your brain a name, e.g., Negative June or Gloom and Doom Bill.)
- Do you have a mechanism that can shut down and reframe the negative self-talk? (For example, when the voice in your head starts sending negative messages, repeat over and over: delete, delete, delete.)
- Do you accept the negative messages literally, without examining whether they are true? (Limit the negative voice to a short, specific amount of time, and imagine putting it in a box or vault.)
- Do you regularly reflect on positive affirmations about who you are? (Remind yourself consistently that you are worthy of being needed and respected.)

8

Positive and Negative Targets

I visualize things in my mind before I have to do them. It is like having a mental workshop.

—Jack Youngblood

At the end of the Vietnam War, prisoners of war, who had been incarcerated for years by the Vietnamese, were released to return to America. Many were in terrible physical shape after the ordeal they had experienced. One pilot had been in a Vietnam prison camp for over six years; nearly 6 feet 3 inches, he weighed slightly less than 100 pounds when he arrived in San Diego. He was dehydrated and had suffered numerous broken bones as a result of beatings; he suffered from malaria and other parasites and, at first observation, had considerable medical challenges that needed to be addressed immediately.

The attending physician, who spent considerable time with the pilot, asked him at one point what was the most immediate thing he would like to happen. Without hesitation, the pilot said, "I would love to play the Torrey Pines golf course." The doctor, a golfer himself, dismissed the request, thinking that he was too weak, and the pilot repeated his request. Incredulous, the doctor responded that walking a golf course was not even remotely possible due to the pilot's condition. The pilot responded, "For more than six years, my captors told me what to do. I thought that was over now that I am home. I would like to play the Torrey Pines golf course tomorrow."

The doctor discussed the situation with his team and decided that he would allow the pilot to go to Torrey Pines in an ambulance, thinking that the pilot would probably take one or two swings, collapse, and be immediately transported back to the hospital. The next morning, when the pilot stepped to the first tee, he drove the ball well over 200 yards down the middle of the fairway. He finished 18 holes of golf and, though dehydrated, was in positive spirits. As he returned to the hospital, the pilot told the medical team over and over about every shot that he had attempted that day. The doctor sat down on his bed, stating, "I am incredulous that you played 18 holes in your condition. I'm a golfer and I know that my physical condition is vastly different from where you are and I am exhausted at the end of the day because of the winds and the challenges of the sand traps. Yet you played 18 holes of golf today. I'm truly amazed. Even more amazing is the fact that you shot 87. But what absolutely blows my mind is that you did not three-putt one green." The pilot smiled and said, "Doc, I haven't three-putted a green in more than six years."

While in captivity the pilot had mentally imagined himself playing golf. In fact, he employed a technique called visualization, a technique that is the foundation for pilots who learn to cope with emergency situations long before they occur. The flyer had literally become an outstanding golfer and an outstanding putter by using a technique that would vitally change the circumstances of his experience. We now know that visualization is critical to outcomes and that human beings and organizations are target oriented. What we see is where we go.

We often hear that a picture is worth a thousand words. That is certainly true with regard to the targets that we set for ourselves. It has been demonstrated, over and over, that the visuals we create for ourselves become the targets for our behavior. The reticular activating system (RAS) in our brain selects opportunities, behaviors, and circumstances that reinforce our ability to achieve the targets we set for ourselves.

Observation and experience have shown that what we say, believe, and see has a tremendous influence on the choices we make in life. For example, the person who is in the market to purchase a new car is well aware, through the media, that the auto dealership is having a sale. In reality, the advertisement announcing the sale has played out hundreds of times over the years, but as the information was not targeted by the brain as important, the brain never noticed it before. Once it became important, the RAS went to work and started to seek out opportunities to fulfill the necessary choices.

If the RAS doesn't get the message that we are leaders, that we choose to be leaders, and that we seek opportunities to lead, the brain will totally ignore resources that make this possible. If we believe we are not leaders, and have visuals that reinforce this belief, the brain will act accordingly.

Critical to the concept of visualization is the development of a scenario in which the individual is already present. For example, when we diet and put photos of ourselves at our heaviest on the refrigerator door, the photos reinforce a negative target. A photo of the person 20 pounds lighter will have a greater consequential effect.

The foundation for behavior is that positive visuals lead to positive outcomes. With regard to leadership, it is imperative to have a positive visual indicating that the desired outcome has already taken place. This visual can be reinforced by positive affirmations:

➤ "I have the skills to be a leader."

➤ "I am capable of making a contribution."

Targets are critical because human beings are visual. What we see has a great deal to do with the choices we make.

Part of the process of authorizing oneself as a leader is to create a series of affirmations and visuals that present the outcome as if it's already happened. If we see ourselves as leaders, the probability that this will happen is greatly enhanced.

Applying Theory to Practice

- Do you see the value of visualization?
- A vision is a magnet. Is yours positive or negative?
- What are your personal and professional targets?
- What are your visuals about leadership?
- If you had a positive visual about leadership, what would its realization feel like?
- Visualize what you would like to happen.
- Visualization enables you to find new resources and people to assist in your goals. What persons and resources are immediately available to you?
- What contributions will you make? Who will benefit the most?

9

The Comfort Zone

Life begins at the end of your comfort zone.

—Neal Donald Wealsh

HOW DOES THE COMFORT ZONE IMPACT LEADERSHIP?

One of the biggest challenges of breaking through boundaries is how to widen one's comfort zone. The comfort zone is the area where individuals feel safe and secure; there are a host of reasons why it's not always easy to step out of one's comfort zone. This complex system is based on feelings, beliefs, successes, failures, and a host of other realities. For example, some people are comfortable speaking in front of a group but others are terrified.

Some opportunities for growth are so daunting and frightening that we reinforce the security of the comfort zone, with affirmations like:

➤ "I could never do that."

➤ "It is impossible for me to do that."

The comfort zone can become a moat around our lives where we decide that there are things we are willing to do and things we are not willing to do.

To move out of one's comfort zone, one must find meaning and leverage. One option is to consciously raise one's level of dissatisfaction with the status quo. Dissatisfaction can be the catalyst that allows us to look for new opportunities and examine new choices, whether significant or insignificant. Dissatisfaction is the foundation, for example, for changing jobs, buying a house, or going to the gym. In all these cases, persons are not satisfied at the conscious or unconscious level, and raising the level of dissatisfaction increases the probability of stepping outside the comfort zone.

This is especially true of leadership. There are a host of examples of how dissatisfaction serves as a catalyst, providing enough energy and inspiration to take some risks. Suppose a person is in a career and feels stuck, believing there is little opportunity to lead. One can accept the situation, complain about it, or be sad about it and continue to stay within the comfort zone. Another choice is to look into the future and ask, "What is the pain of having nothing change or of staying right where I am now?" Still another option is to reframe the question in a positive way by asking, "What is the pleasure of looking at the situation differently?" "How could I further my opportunities either within this organization or elsewhere?" The level of dissatisfaction is the foundation for new choices. Thus, cultivating dissatisfaction is not necessarily a negative phenomenon. If we see that we have come to a point where we do not want to be, then dissatisfaction can promote alternatives.

HOW DOES ONE START TO MOVE OUT OF THE COMFORT ZONE?

Some leadership opportunities are so compelling that it is possible to take a large leap out of the comfort zone. An example is to lead the accreditation team within a school of nursing; the project is impactful, has organizational visibility, and has the potential for future promotional rewards. However, when the incentives are not so apparent, it is probably wise to gently start to move out of the comfort zone.

Dissatisfaction is the foundation because it clearly delineates why there is reason to take steps to move out of the comfort zone. Listing all the reasons why dissatisfaction is present enables a person to more clearly understand the price of staying within their comfort zone. There is always going to be some level of discomfort, of not being sure that this is the right direction. If the dissatisfaction is strong enough with a positive visual, then leaving the comfort zone and behaving differently will probably make sense.

Applying Theory to Practice

- What would give you leverage to start to move gingerly out of your comfort zone?
- What is your level of dissatisfaction regarding leadership opportunities?
- Is it strong enough to promote change?
- What pain will you feel in the future if you do not move out of your comfort zone?
- What is the pleasure you will experience by moving out of your comfort zone?
- Should I raise my level of dissatisfaction? How would I accomplish this?

10

Failure and Rejection

It is fine to celebrate success but it is more important to heed the lessons of failure.

—Bill Gates

DO PAST FAILURES RULE OUT LEADERSHIP?

Anthony had a significant failure in his department seven years ago; for reasons beyond his control, his department was over budget on the development of a new product. Since that time his belief that he is a failure has affected him on every level of his being. He lives with a high degree of guilt and has been hesitant to take on any project that is risky. He fears rejection, and work, which once was a vital source of fulfillment, has become a place where he is simply marking time until retirement.

Failure and rejection form a tough boundary that threatens sense of self and meaning and inhibits growth and development. Most human beings carry with them the scar tissue of past failures at an intense level or as a series of mistakes made along the way. The baggage of failure is a reality that often keeps us from selecting new behaviors and opportunities. Those who have not failed at anything have probably led a reclusive life, as failure is part and parcel of the human experience.

In our quest for leadership, we as authors have no pretense of not having failed at certain things. Each time a person sets out on a new path there is always the risk that it will not go well, and that is certainly true of leadership. As we have mentioned before, leadership can be messy, difficult, and painful, but we believe that in the final analysis, it is one of the most wonderful experiences for personal and professional fulfillment.

It is not prudent to ignore failure or treat it as trivial. Rather failure is, in a very real sense, an opportunity for learning. What are the circumstances in which the failure occurred? Are we doomed to repeat failure? Will failure always influence the choices we make in the present and the future? It is important to examine the experience of failure and to ask how we would behave differently if given the chance. Failure only becomes a life sentence if we avoid examining failure and rejection and believe there are no future opportunities.

Applying Theory to Practice

- Is rejection or failure blocking your ability to lead?
- Are you avoiding opportunities because you are afraid to fail?
- Have you rationally examined your past failures?
- Does failure limit your ability to take reasonable risks?
- Describe your biggest fears. What is the worst thing that could happen?
- Is there a distinction in your mind between "I have failed" and "I am a failure"?
- What would be the first steps you would consider taking if you were to move beyond your fear of rejection?
- Where can you find leverage to begin the process?
- What is your current attitude toward rejection and failure?
- Can you depersonalize your past failures and not let them own your current choices?

The Lone Ranger

11

Even the Lone Ranger did not do it alone.

—Harvey MacKay

Rachel has observed that the most successful people in her organization seem to have a high degree of intelligence, are quick to act, and rely more on themselves than on anyone else. This is somewhat of a handicap for Rachel because she is aware that there are areas in which she would love to grow and develop but she has no experience. She's come to the conclusion that perhaps she is not as qualified to be a leader as she initially hoped because, she realizes, there are areas in her skill bank that need supplemental help. She believes that she has an inherent weakness and is incapable of developing the necessary skills for leadership. In essence, she has assumed the Lone Ranger approach to leadership, believing that she has to be all-knowing and fully competent in all areas before she attempts to assume a position of leadership.

One of the more consequential boundaries to leadership is the belief that as leaders, we must be competent in all areas and able to perform all tasks with certitude and strength. Our observation over the years is that trying to lead as the Lone Ranger is almost always a surefire way to burn out. The Lone Ranger will never achieve the level of success that is possible with the aid of mentors, allies, and stakeholders. It is not necessary for leaders to be isolated or to take the position that requesting aid or assistance is somehow a weakness.

Leadership is not an isolated venture. Rather, it is the understanding that bringing people together achieves outcomes that could not be fulfilled by any one individual. The posture of perfection is also not helpful because it is not possible. The search for excellence is more vital because it can be achieved by using all the resources that are available. Individuals do not rise and fall as leaders solely based on individual skills. No one has the ability to answer all questions or challenges in isolation. It is critical as leaders to seek allies who not only support us, but who challenge us to raise the bar, provide valuable feedback, and provide support, especially in those moments when leadership becomes messy and difficult.

Applying Theory to Practice

- Do you have a mentor or mentors?
- What are the areas that you need to develop?
- Do you have a network? If so, are you actively involved with those in your network?
- How would you go about seeking a mentor in your network?
- What prevents you from seeking a mentor's assistance?
- Do you have any allies in your organization?
- Do you need further educational or coaching assistance?
- Do you believe that you should invest in yourself at this time?
- Are there any current training or educational opportunities for your development?
- Do you need to invest time and add resources to your skillset?

12

Setting Specific Positive Goals

Goals are the fuel in the furnace of achievement.

—Brian Tracy

There is a wonderful moment in *Alice's Adventures in Wonderland* by Lewis Carroll when Alice has a choice to make about direction. She has to make a choice about two roads, and she asks the Cheshire cat which direction she should take. This question is met with a response from the Cheshire cat: "That depends a good deal on where you want to go." Alice replies, "I don't much care where." And the cat answers, "Then it doesn't matter which way you go."

There are many times in our lives when we live on the Island of Someday. We look at our circumstances and challenges and tell ourselves that someday we will do something about this. However, for many, someday never happens. It is not a question of insincerity—we would really like to have this happen. We think about the outcome we desire, and that provides a warm feeling that is often dissipated by the realities and activities of life. So, in a sense, we wish certain things will happen and want them to happen, but our desires do not have the strength of choice and action.

One way to address this positively is to create a specific goal-setting process. It is important to specify, in behavioral terms, what our specific goals look like. The more definition that is brought to the goal, the higher the probability the goal will be achieved. If a person verbally mentions a desired goal, the probability of achieving the goal is somewhere around 4 percent. If the person writes it down, the probability of achieving the goal moves to somewhere around 40 percent. Writing the goal down, signing the paper, and starting to develop a plan to achieve the goal moves the needle to approximately 60 percent. Writing it down, signing the paper, creating a plan, naming a specific date to complete the goal, and inviting someone to help monitor progress moves the needle to about 90 percent that the goal will be achieved (Canfield, 2015).

Goal setting is not a miracle process. It requires consistent focus and actionable behaviors. The process of setting specific measurable goals is a way to break through the boundaries that prevent successful completion of goals. Goal setting provides a visual target with not only the opportunity to see the target but to move toward it in concrete ways. There will be adjustments, and additional resources may be required, but those who follow this process will be stunned by the remarkable results they achieve.

Applying Theory to Practice

- What are your specific goals for leadership?
- Will you write them down, assign a date for each goal, and sign the document?
- What would be the immediate next steps?
- Who can assist you in the process?
- Can you see the finished state and feel the feelings that will accompany the attainment of your goals?

13

Diversity: Reality Check

Strength lies in differences, not in similarities.

—Stephen R. Covey

Andy, a human resources recruiter, has been working with Robert, a manager who is interviewing candidates for an assistant manager's position. Mustafa, an applicant, has not received any information about his status. Andy contacts Robert because he is concerned that it has been more than three weeks and Mustafa hasn't been contacted. He has concerns about the hiring process and asks if Mustafa is still a viable candidate. Robert states that he needs to hire someone quickly and with skills. Andy had reviewed Mustafa's resume and reminds Robert that Mustafa has held a similar position and is well qualified. Robert indicates that he feels more comfortable with the two other candidates because has worked with them before (the two in-house applicants are a white male and a white female). Andy assures Robert that if he interviewed Mustafa, he might have a different opinion. Robert responds that he is concerned that Mustafa does not speak English well and may not be able to understand him. When Andy reminds Robert about the company's nondiscrimination policy, Robert says that he is aware and has participated in diversity training but this situation does not apply. He will not interview Mustafa because it would be a waste of time.

There are many forms of diversity in society, for example, race, ethnicity, gender, sexual orientation and gender identity, socioeconomic status, age, disabilities, religious beliefs, political beliefs, and other attributes (NLN, 2016). Corporations have made much progress over the past 10 years in opening doors and establishing more inviting and inclusive environments for lesbian, gay, bisexual, transgender (LBGT) employees. However, some employees will not reveal their sexual identity because of their "system in the mind," the belief they will be ostracized—and in some companies that will happen (Hewlett & Sumberg, 2011, 1–2).

According to Hewlett and Yoshino (2016), LGBT-inclusive companies are better at three things that make them more competitive in hiring diverse employees and gaining market share for their products: these companies excel in attracting and retaining top talent, gaining recognition from other companies, and winning the business and loyalty of discerning consumers.

Although the literature indicates that men in nontraditional professions, such as nursing, may experience discrimination in the workplace, they also on occasion receive preferential treatment (McMurray, 2011). Women, on the other hand, typically experience discrimination in the workplace, and for black women and other women of color, the issues having to do with gender and leadership are compounded. Society, even today, has biases about women's ability to be leaders and their ability to hold top-level positions in organizations, such as CEOs.

In some family systems, these biases begin during childhood with differentiation between male and female children—how they are treated and the toys they are given. Subtle messages are sent, either consciously or unconsciously. Also operating consciously or unconsciously is the "system in the mind," which refers to biases, stereotypes, assumptions, perceptions, and experiences that may influence behaviors toward others.

The "system in the mind" shapes the gender biases women encounter. Research has demonstrated that due to stereotypes there is a difference in how female and male leaders are perceived and expected to behave (Eagly, Karen, & Makhijani, 1995) with women and men more successful in leadership roles aligned with their gender. Primarily, men are indoctrinated to be assertive, decisive, independent, and strategic, while women are expected to be caring, compassionate, and nurturing (Brandt & Laiho, 2013; Hoyt, Simm, & Reid, 2009). These perceptions of women leaders can have negative ramifications that influence their ability to lead others. The expectations may also impact whether or not a woman is promoted; the perception may be that women do not have the capability to lead in certain positions. This way of thinking places limitations on women and their ability to be successful and climb the career ladder.

Diversity biases exist at the system level as well as the individual level. The organizational culture may perpetuate stereotypes and biases and fail to promote diversity and inclusion. Thus, this puts women leaders, especially women of color, at a disadvantage. However, all is not gloom and doom. There must be a systems change in policies and practices, support for women, the development of women leaders, and the creation of internal and external networks. There must be visible career pathways for promotion in organizations.

This process cannot be a secret; there must be transparency. Finally, these changes have to be co-created with all women leaders in the organization.

According to Clayton (2010), many companies have integrated diversity programs but use the promotion of women and people of color as the only success metric: "So, the challenge looks something like this: Having diversity, while inevitable, does not automatically bring harmony, success and profitability. In fact, it can cause more problems if the difference in values, cultures and behaviors are not effectively managed. With the increasing importance of intellectual and human capital on organizational success, managing the increasing diversity of today's global workforce is a critical enabler for all successful organizations" (p. 2).

Women leaders have an integral role in co-creating change. They need to find their personal power within themselves to lead in their roles. They must act in a way that shows them belonging in their positions. Women leaders must realize they are not imposters, because they are competent and have the capability to lead. They must free themselves from the boundaries in their minds that hold them hostage because they deserve to be at the table and have their voices heard. This reminds me of one of McBride's (2015) developmental tensions of leadership: "finding your authoritative voice versus giving voice to others" (327). It means that as women leaders move through their career trajectory, they must be able to find their voices to lead and at the same time, help others to find their voices to lead. The microphone must be passed around so that there are many voices, perhaps sometimes singing the same tune or sometimes singing a different tune. Women leaders must realize they are not alone because for effective transformation to occur there has to be a partnership. The system must allow them to lead successfully across internal and external boundaries.

If negative boundaries are removed, and companies become more committed to diversity and inclusion, then the baton for Roving Leadership can be passed to individuals representing all types of diversity. And organizations can take advantage of robust leadership skills that diverse employees bring to the table. While diversity in the workplace can lead to challenges and situations that may become difficult to resolve, today's workforce calls for all types of diversity.

One type of diversity that is sometimes easy to overlook in the workplace is diversity of thinking styles. According to Miller (2014), there are benefits of diversity of thought that include "a clearer perspective for a broad audience segment — Your target markets and audiences are diverse and made up of the full gamut of thinking and behavioral styles; utilize in-house resources to ensure communication is on point across the board" (2). Following are some advantages of diversity of thinking:

> *Creative tension:* With diversity in thinking styles, the creative process becomes a more combative formula, in a good way. The best ideas result, usually as a combination of many perspectives.

> *Employee engagement:* When employees know their thinking and behavioral styles are appreciated, engagement increases, along with the propensity to contribute.

> *Appreciation of all kinds of diversity:* When cognitive diversity is touted and appreciated, employees see that differences go beyond attributes such as culture, race, gender, and experience. They understand that these, too, must be valued.

> *Speed to proficiency:* With a cognitively diverse workforce, employees can more easily find those who think and behave in their preferred format. They accentuate their strengths to become more proficient more quickly.

Diverse individuals must create positive affirmations such as the following:

> Acknowledge your accomplishments. You've worked hard to get where you are.

> You deserve to be in your current position. Become self-authorized to lead.

> Don't compete with others; compete with yourself. Become greater than great.

> Be comfortable in your own skin.

> Being perfect is a myth. There are no perfect people. Perfection is an illusion.

> Engage in positive self-talk so that the messages you hear in your mind become an automatic response.

> Don't allow others to marginalize you.

> Be confident, but not arrogant.

> Follow your dreams and aspirations.

> Don't hide out and become invisible.

> Change negative self-talk to positive self-talk.

> Buy into your value as a person and the value you bring to the company.

> Don't collude with the system against you and others.

Applying Theory to Practice

- Do you have the "imposter syndrome"? If so, write down your reasons.
- Identify the things in your "system in the mind" that are holding you hostage.
- What are your fears?
- Identify one positive experience you've had in your current position.
- Identify one negative experience you've had in your current position. What were lessons learned?
- To what extent do you feel valued as a leader in your organization?
- How can you influence changes in your organization's culture, if appropriate?
- Take up your own authority to be a leader.
- Do not buy into others' stereotypes and biases of you.

14

Introverts Versus Extroverts

In a gentle way you can shake the world.

—Mahatma Ghandi

Connie joined a Fortune 500 pharmaceutical company as the executive director for human resources reporting to the vice president for human resources. After eight months on the job, working long hours, she was eager to prove her competence, please her boss, and develop relationships with those individuals with whom she felt comfortable. The organization was committed to a culture of collaboration, team work, working across silos, openness to new ideas, and best practices. Equally important was a culture of diversity by gender and ethnicity. One evening while working late, Connie's boss/mentor stopped by her office for a chat. "Happy to have you here. You are working hard but working hard at the wrong thing. You are working hard at the work rather than building relationships. Relationships help you get work done with and through the people." The boss/mentor told Connie that she wasn't getting help in executing her vision of "HR becoming a strategic partner in the business." He told her that she needed to "change her behavior and SHOW UP."

Connie's behavior of "not showing up" was based on her very low need to be inclusive of and participate with others. She invited others but did not engage with others when invited and had a high preference for introversion. Specifically, Connie worked alone and independently; had a need for privacy; was sometimes quiet and difficult to read; and while she was talkative in areas in which she had a lot of knowledge, that happened only with close friends. Connie accepted her supervisor's comments and began to change her behavior. She ate lunch with others in the cafeteria as well as at restaurants; built relationships appropriately with others; and engaged her staff in co-creating HR's vision aligned with the organization. She learned several lessons, and realized that failure to modify her behavior would hinder her effectiveness in creating a broad network, opening herself to different perspectives, building and maintaining relationships, and developing an understanding and appreciation of different styles. She realized she had the ability to modify her behavior and act as an extrovert in certain situations, returning to her comfort zone as an introvert in the confines of her home. Connie remained with the company for eight successful years.

Carl Jung (1921) identified two psychological traits: introvert and extrovert. The introvert's focus is internal, whereas extroverts are focused on the external world and the people who surround them. Jung identified these traits in accordance with one's relationship to objects and one's worldview. The introvert's lens has a more subjective quality, whereas the extrovert looks through the lens based on objective data. Jung cautioned about not being aware of individual differences, which would influence how one functions as an introvert or extrovert. He postulated that these psychological traits are on a continuum and all individuals may have both traits with one trait being more dominant.

Jung's psychological traits were the basis of the development of the Meyers-Briggs test, a personality traits assessment instrument that is widely used in organizations.

Some traits (Cain, 2012; Jung, 1921) of extroverts include:

> Has the ability to make decisions based on facts; doesn't deal well with the abstract.

> Is outgoing and sociable.

> Works well in groups, but may have some difficulty when others are not in agreement with one's ideas.

> May move into situations without careful thinking.

> Gets energy from engaging with large groups.

Some traits (Cain, 2012; Jung, 1921) of introverts include:

> Likes solitude and personal space.

> Is a good listener.

> Is analytical.

> Is shy, possibly due to an underlying fear of social situations.

> Is calm, cautious, and deliberate.

Susan Cain, author of the book *Quiet: The Power of Introverts in a World that Can't Stop Talking* (2012), stated in an interview with the *Guardian* (2012) that "[I]ntroverts prefer lower-stimulation environments, that's where they feel at their most alive. Whereas extroverts really crave stimulation in order to feel at their best. It's important to see it this way because people often equate introversion with being antisocial, and it's not that at all—it's just a preference."

In society, there are stereotypes and biases about introverts and extroverts that tend toward a negative view. Introverts are forced to live in a sea of extroverts, and what becomes important is how they manage the waves and ensure that there is a lifeboat when it's needed. Introverts can be said to have quiet power or quiet strength because they have the power of adaptability when the occasion arises for them to change their behavior, leave their comfort zone, and function as extroverts.

The introvert has the ability to be a chameleon. Think of playing hide and seek—now you see me and now you don't. Introverted leaders must be aware that there are times they need to be seen and heard. It is important to note that introverts can be excellent leaders. For example, the Reverend Martin Luther King Jr., Mother Teresa, and Rosa Parks, some of our greatest leaders, were introverts. It's about adaptability and stepping up to lead.

In identifying leadership strategies for introverts, Sherman (2013) uses the term *ambivert,* first *identified by* psychologist Hans Eysenck in 1947 as a personality type between introvert and extrovert. For Sherman, ambiverts have the ability to take on the characteristics of both an introvert and extrovert. They are more flexible, more intuitive, and more influential.

As you lead as an extrovert, introvert, or ambivert, it is important to remember that leadership is not lodged in one single individual. Thus, you have a great opportunity to engage the team in solutions, carrying out tasks and allowing others to take up their authority to lead alongside you.

Applying Theory to Practice

Sherman (2013) identified the following strategies for introverted leaders to maximize their potential:

- Recognize there isn't anything wrong with you.
- Celebrate your successes.
- Be cautious about the leadership opportunities you select. It may be better sometimes to choose those that require less social interaction and more immersion in your work (if you have a choice).
- Intentionally create time in your schedule to reactivate your energy.
- Remember that there may be times when you have to push yourself to interact with people in the organization.
- Delegate some activities that are taxing to extroverted members of the team.
- Be aware that you can become so immersed in a project that you lose sight of the time, which may impact completion of other tasks.
- Learn to be adaptable and become self-authorized to lead.

15

Microinequities: To Tell the Truth

Micro-inequities are subtle, often unconscious, messages that devalue, discourage and impair workplace performance.

—Eric L. Hinton and Stephen Young

A beautiful 23-year-old biracial woman is struggling with her heritage and her identify. Her mother is Italian and Cuban and her father is black. She finds that she must be dealing with microinequities through micromessaging but does not know what she is experiencing—just that it does not make her feel good about herself. The micromessages became so powerful that she decides to depict them in a picture. She draws a young, beautiful woman with long, flowing black hair, with her face in three geometric pieces—one with a light brown complexion, one with a medium brown complexion, and the last a darker shade of brown. In the young woman's hair, she names the microinequities she has experienced:

- You're black.
- So exotic.
- You're lying.
- Do you speak Spanish?
- You must be Indian.
- Where are your parents from?
- I knew you had some Spanish in you.
- That's a sexy mix.
- But you don't look like it.
- What are you?

The experience of microaggression can be devastating for young people who are dealing with issues of identity in a world where others want them to be something or someone else, based on their stereotypes and biases. In 1973, Mary Rowe (2008) coined the term "micro-inequities" when working for the chancellor of the Massachusetts Institute of Technology in efforts to identify ways to improve the workplace for underrepresented groups, for example, men and women of color, white women, and people with disabilities. The term is applied to persons of various religious groups and in comments about age, sexual orientation, gender identity, and political beliefs. Rowe described microinequities as "apparently small events, which are often ephemeral and hard-to-prove, events, which are covert, often unintentional, frequently unrecognized by the perpetrator, which occur whenever people are perceived to be different" (2).

The micromessages that evolve from microinequities can be gestures, signs of indifference such as blank looks and other nonverbal behaviors, and the discounting of experiences or comments (Rowe, 2008; Young, 2010). Young writes: "In a 10-minute conversation, we send between 40 and 150 micro-messages. Each day, we typically send 2,000 and 4,000 positive or negative micro-messages" (2010, 1).

Sometimes microinequities are so subtle that the person on the receiving end is not quite aware of what just happened, aside from having a strange and uncomfortable feeling that something is not right. It is only upon reflection about the situation, or processing the experience with someone else, that the realization of what has happened comes to the forefront.

Microinequities can have a devastating impact on the individual as well as the company or institution. Individuals can be left feeling incompetent and devalued, with a lack of self-confidence and self-worth. Organizationally, there may be a decrease in morale and job satisfaction. Rowe (2008) and Young (2010) state that the best way to manage microinequities is with transparency and open discussion in the organization.

Young (2017) presented a third concept: microadvantages. These are subtle, usually unconscious, messages that inspire, motivate, and enhance workplace performance. Tone of voice and verbal and nonverbal messages are positive. When applied effectively, microadvantages can unleash resources and strengths in individuals to maximize their potential.

Finally, it is important to recognize action steps to use in organizations to address microinequities:

▸ Recognize when employees are experiencing microinequities.

▸ Be aware when we may be sending micromessages.

▸ Establish an organizational culture that doesn't tolerate microinequities.

▸ Honor and celebrate differences.

▸ Apprise management that microinequities are occurring in the organization.

In organizations, it takes commitment and collective action to eliminate microinequities. There must be awareness and acknowledgement that they exist and a willingness to confront issues intentionally and consistently.

Applying Theory to Practice

- Describe your experience with microinequities. What did you do?
- Who did you talk to about the situation(s)?
- Was there any resolution?
- Were you able to find your voice to have a crucial conversation with the person?
- If you continue to experience microinequities, with what official in your organization would you discuss this situation?
- Identify strategies you will use in the future when you experience microinequities.

16

Putting It All Together

The only walls that exist are those you have placed in your mind. And whatever obstacles you conceive, exist only because you have forgotten what you have already achieved.

—Suzy Kassem

Roving Leadership is about being aware of the boundaries, both positive and negative, that are discussed in this book. These barriers may confront us on a daily basis. Once we are able to identify what we are experiencing, we can begin to develop intentional strategies to manage them and/or capitalize on them. This will help us become better leaders.

A critical misunderstanding we often have with regard to leadership is that true leadership exists only when the consequences are monumental. In fact, leadership opportunities appear often during the course of a normal day. Authorizing oneself to respond is at the heart of Roving Leadership.

Great moments in life happen when we act on the belief and conviction that we are leaders. We do not need permission before authorizing ourselves to act as leaders. Each one of us has skills and talents, a unique voice and style, and we all deserve to have leadership opportunities. Once this belief becomes operational, we will find opportunities to lead that are readily within our reach.

To take the step toward achieving our leadership goals, we must examine and reject the barriers that block our way. Leadership is not a one-size-fits-all phenomenon. It can be taught, and no one style is better than another. One individual may be verbal or extroverted and lead, while another, who is shy or introverted, can lead as well. It is wise to select a style of leadership that is consistent with who we are. Authenticity is more important than any particular style.

Being an authentic leader leads to trust and honesty. It creates a positive organizational culture where people want to become engaged in implementing the organization's goals. Individuals feel valued by the leader and want to maximize their ability to perform. Collective engagement becomes important for innovation as well as individual and organizational transformation. All individuals flourish and the organization as a whole becomes more sustainable because it is operating at its best, with multiple instances of Roving Leadership.

Leadership will not always be easy and, at times, some of us may feel stuck, without options, and even wonder whether what we are doing has value. At these moments it is imperative to adhere to the belief that regardless of the circumstances, there are always choices.

As we pursue our desire to lead, the voices in our head may spew out negative self-talk and self-limiting beliefs. We can limit the effect of these phenomena by refusing to accept their validity and by substituting positive self-talk and widening supportive beliefs. Rational reflection and the examination of feelings lead to choice and constructive ways to move beyond our comfort zone.

Failure and rejection will only own us if the fear of stumbling once again is allowed to keep us from moving out of our comfort zone. Our initial attempts may be small, but our new behaviors are a way of creating new leadership opportunities.

All of this is enhanced by the creation of positive visuals that become the magnets of the conscious and subconscious mind. We are all are target oriented, and what we see, say, and believe creates a platform for constructive growth and development.

To achieve the Roving Leadership success we desire, we must resist the temptation to go it alone. We all need allies and mentors to assist us. The desire to add helpers is a sign of strength, not weakness. It is also essential to invest in ourselves by taking advantage of educational and experiential opportunities to develop new skills.

Organizations that are aware of barriers such as diversity issues and systemic microinequities must position leaders to examine the source of these issues and engage in courageous conversations, avoiding the temptation to respond with lip service and engage in platitudes. It is important to develop policies about what is acceptable in how people are treated, especially those who may be different with regard to age, gender identity, sexual orientation, religion, and disability. Leaders in organizations should explore their own "system in the mind," which can potentially affect hiring and promotion opportunities for women and ethnic and religious minorities. Leaders must determine how they want to integrate the concept of Roving Leadership in their organizations for the benefit of equal opportunity and transformation. By taking these actions, those overlooked for leadership positions may emerge as leaders.

Finally, specific goal setting is the foundation for implementing Roving Leadership and for achieving future and current success. Specify your leadership goals by writing them down, noting specific dates for meeting goals, and signing the paper. Create a plan for each goal and ask someone to monitor your progress.

The theory of Roving Leadership is based on empirical evidence that with the right set of circumstances and challenges, everyone can be a leader. Regardless of the environment, there are opportunities to make a difference. Roving Leadership is a framework for transforming individuals and the organization by widening the concept of leadership. The foundation is shared power, responsibilities, and accountability within the organization. Once all individuals understand that their contributions are vital to the organization and receive recognition for their contributions, the culture will be transformed.

The job of leadership is not merely to sell a view or a goal, but to enroll others in creating value and sharing risk. By advocating and supporting Roving Leadership, organizations and individuals discover their strengths and, it is hoped, change for the better.

There is a nexus between boundaries and Roving Leadership. If leaders do not address for themselves the boundaries discussed in this book, they cannot be mentally free to become Roving Leaders themselves, nor will they have the ability to assist others on their team or in the organization to engage in the process. Leaders in organizations must commit to addressing boundaries effectively so that the leadership of others in the organization is enhanced.

Let's summarize the benefits of Roving Leadership for the organization:

> It allows different voices to be heard.

> It invites individuals to assume their own authority to lead and supports them in the process.

> It leads to strategies to deal with complexity and allows innovation to flourish.

> And most important, by allowing for a kaleidoscope of diverse leaders, with different ways of thinking, it creates conditions that encourage others to take up their own authority to lead. A kaleidoscope of leaders is needed today to make sense of the chaos of systems and unleash a world of untapped resources.

We invite you to give yourself permission to take off the mask—to have the vision to break through boundaries and the courage to lead with your core values intact, your own North Star. Now you're ready to embark on the Roving Leadership journey!

References

Bennis, W. (2009). *On becoming a leader.* New York, NY: Basic Books.

Bolman, L. G., & Deal, T. E. (2013). *Reframing organizations: Artistry, choices, and leadership* (8th ed.). San Francisco, CA: Jossey-Bass.

Brandt, T., & Laiho, M. (2013). Gender and personality in transformational leadership: An examination of leaders and subordinates' perspective. *Leadership and Organizational Development Journal, 34*(1), 46–66.

Cain, S. (2012). *Quiet: The power of introverts in a world where people can't stop talking.* New York, NY: Random House.

Cain, S. (2012). Society has a cultural bias towards extroverts. *The Guardian.* Retrieved from https://www.theguardian.com/technology/2012/apr/01/susan-cain-extrovert-introvert-interview

Canfield (2015). Workshop in the Quantum Lead program, Philadelphia, March 2015.

Carroll, L. (n.d.). Lewis Carroll Quotes. Retrieved from www.goodreads.com/quotes/815118-i-knew-who-i-was-this-morning-but-i-ve-changed

Clayton Sr., C. B. (2010). *The diversity profit equation* [Corporate White Paper]. Retrieved from https://www.ithaca.edu/hr/docs/other/attach/EC2014_CC_WP_DQ.pdf

Eagly, A. H., Karan, S. J., & Makhijani, M. G. (1995). Gender and the effectiveness of leaders manage: A meta-analysis. *Psychological Bulletin, 1117*, 125–145.

Frankl, V. E. (1959). *Man's search for meaning.* New York, NY: Simon & Schuster.

Hewlett, S., & Sumberg, K. (2011, July-August). For LGBT workers, being "out" bring advantages. *Harvard Business Review.* Retrieved from https://hbr.org/2011/07/for-lgbt-workers-being-out-brings-advantages

Hewlett, S., & Yoshino, K. (2016). LGBT-Inclusive companies are better at 3 big things. *Harvard Business Review.* Retrieved from https://hbr.org/2016/02/lgbt-inclusive-companies-are-better-at-3-big-things

Hinton, E. L. Micro-inequities: When small slights lead to huge problems in the workplace. Diversity Inc. Magazine. March/April 2003. Princeton, NJ: Diversity Inc. Media LLC.

Hoyt, C. L., Simm, S., & Reid, L. (2009). Choosing the best wo(man) for the job: The effects of mortality, sex and gender and gender stereotypes on leader evaluation. *The Leadership Quarterly, 20*(2), 233–243.

Jung, C. G. (1921). *Psychological types: General description of the types.* Translation by Bayes, H. G. (1923) in *Classics in the history of psychology.* An internet resource developed by Green, C. G. York University, Toronto, Ontario. http://psychclassics.yorku.ca/Jung/types.htm

Kotter, J. P. (2012). *Leading change.* Boston, MA: Harvard Business Review.

McBride, A. B. (2015). Leading-following perspectives. *Nursing Science Quarterly, 33*(4), 326–329.

McMurray, T. (2011). The image of male nurses and nursing leadership mobility. *Nursing Forum, 46*(1), 22–28. doi:10.1111/j.1744-6198.2010.00206.x

Miller, M. (2014). *Want results? Look to diversity in thinking styles* [Web log post]. Retrieved from www.emergenetics.com/blog/results-diversity-thinking-styles/

National League for Nursing. (2016). Achieving diversity and meaningful inclusion in nursing education. [NLN Vision Series]. Retrieved from http://www.nln.org/docs/default-source/about/vision-statement-achieving-diversity.pdf?sfvrsn=2

Rowe, M. (2008). Micro-affirmations and micro-inequities. *Journal of International Ombudsman Association, 1*(1).

Sherman, R. (2013). Introverts can be nurse leaders too. *American Nurse Today, 34*(8), 1–3.

Young, S. (2010, March 29). Micro-inequities: The power of small. *The Junction. Diversity and Inclusion Newsletter,* 16th edition.

Young, S. (2017). *Micromessaging: Why great leadership is beyond words.* New York: McGraw Hill Education.

Walumbwa, F., Avolio, B., Gardner, W., Wernsing, T., & Peterson, S. (2008). Authentic leadership: Development and validation of a theory-based measure. *Journal of Management, 34*(1), 89–126. Retrieved from http://digitalcommons. unl.edu/cgi/viewcontent.cgi?article= 1021&context=managementfacpub. doi:10.1177/0149206307308913